Relapse F
Bipolar D

A treatment r

workbook for therapist and client

Relapse Prevention in Bipolar Disorder

A treatment manual and
workbook for therapist and client

Dr John Sorensen

UNIVERSITY OF
HERTFORDSHIRE PRESS

First published in Great Britain in 2005 by
University of Hertfordshire Press
Learning and Information Services
University of Hertfordshire
College Lane
Hatfield
Hertfordshire AL10 9AB

British Library Cataloguing in Publication Data
A catalogue record for this book is available from the British Library

ISBN 1-902806-56-5 paperback manual plus 5 workbooks
ISBN 1-902806-57-3 pack of 10 workbooks sold separately

Designed by Geoff Green, Cambridge CB4 5RA
Cover designed by John Robertshaw, Harpenden AL5 2JB
Printed in Great Britain by Antony Rowe Ltd, Chippenham SN14 6LH

Every man is in a ravine alone.
His solitude and this ravine are his
problem, they are also his sanctuary.

Ralph Maynard Smith

Comments about the Sorensen Therapy for Instability in Mood from clinicians

"The manual and the intervention it describes are likely to have a significant impact on the lives of people diagnosed as suffering from bipolar disorder, and to be of considerable value to clinicians working in mental health settings."

Professor David Winter, Head of Clinical Psychology Services (Barnet), Barnet, Enfield and Haringey Mental Health NHS Trust

"This new therapy appears at a point in time when it is most needed ... it has become clear that bipolar affective disorder is much more prevalent in the psychiatric population than previously known ... The Sorensen Therapy for Instability in Mood will make it possible for the majority of patients, outside of the university clinics, to benefit from effective treatment. To my knowledge there are no other such programmes available."

Dr Jens-Emil Viftrup, Consultant Psychiatrist, Adult Mental Health

"The therapy developed by Sorensen ... is likely to be of significant value to clients who crave a sense of understanding and control over a 'disorder' that so often severely disrupts their lives on many levels. His innovative psychological therapy provides a much-needed augmentation to the often unilateral (and predominantly medical) treatment currently available to those given a diagnosis of 'bipolar disorder' ... Both the thorough and systematic description of the therapy in the manual, and the relapse prevention resource it provides to clients, will help professionals and clients alike feel quickly confident in applying this new approach ... which will enable those who live with the effects of severe mood instability to develop a sense of renewed agency and hope."

Dr Maria Gennoy, Consultant Clinical Psychologist

"I recommend wholly John Sorensen's therapeutic method and believe that it will be of interest to practitioners."

John Rhodes, Consultant Clinical Psychologist, Joint Head of Adult Mental Health (Haringey) and Honorary Lecturer at University College London

"Such a brief but effective intervention would undoubtedly be a significant contribution to the psychological treatment of [bipolar disorder]."

Graham Huff, Head of Psychological Services, Chadwick Lodge, Milton Keynes

Comments from clients who have undergone the treatment

"I feel a lot more confident … It's understanding it now, more … Someone's taken time out to explain it bit by bit … and to know that when I start feeling something there is a reason behind that, and to delve a bit deeper and find out what the reason was in the first place. And then use the treatment to change it. I feel a lot more confident because I know a lot more … I think why I found this [treatment] particularly useful is as a way to get to the deeper stuff, like you are making choices about things you can do, you can act on … I can make those choices … I feel different about it, I feel hopeful, really."

"My mother would know that something was up straight away but I could never talk to her. Whereas I have a brilliant relationship with my mother now. She's read [the workbook] … It's helped her … She has seen, since I've had this treatment, a completely different person come out. I'm a lot happier."

"[The treatment] has broken down the illness into bite-size, manageable pieces, that has allowed me to digest what it is to be ill like me."

"It worked wonders … It is very good … I do really think I will use it again. I think it is important to keep it because you just forget little things and it is the little things that count."

"This was definitely the most useful and applicable thing, so thank you."

Contents

Acknowledgements

Special thanks go to the participants in the study validating the present intervention. All of the participants stayed committed to the project and made valuable comments on the treatment, which have been taken into account in the current manual.

I would also like to thank Dr John Done and Jane Housham, University of Hertfordshire, who both saw the potential of the treatment at an early stage and gave generously of their time.

Finally, I would like to thank my partner Kathryn Smith without whose support and advice this treatment would never have come about.

Dr John Sorensen
North Manchester General Hospital

Introduction

Bipolar disorder (BPD) is a debilitating, typically recurring and severe mental illness often occurring with serious secondary consequences in the form of suicidal behaviours, physical health problems and substance abuse (Goodwin and Jamison, 1990; Michalak, Yatham and Lam, 2004; Scott and Todd, 2002). It is also clear that these problems are frequently confounded by impairments in occupational and social functioning more generally and that these impairments persist even when symptom relief has been achieved for a given person with BPD (Coryell et al., 1993; Dion, Tohen, Anthony and Waternaux, 1988; Tohen et al., 2003).

The standard treatment offered to patients remains prophylactic pharmacological interventions and a range of medications are being used with some success (Geddes, Burgess, Hawton, Jamison and Guy, 2004). However, using the medical approach in isolation has significant limitations at both symptomatic and functional levels, as illustrated by limited long-term effectiveness and non-adherence (Greenhouse, Meyer and Johnson, 2000; Huxley, 2002; Keck, McElroy, Strakowski, Bourne and West, 1997; Kessler, Rubinow, Holmes, Abelson and Zhao, 1997; Nilsson, 1999). For example, one longitudinal study reported a relapse risk of 37 per cent after one year and 73 per cent after five or more years for patients on continual mood-stabilising medication (Gitlin, Swendsen, Heller and Hammen, 1995). Such findings illustrate the need for a biopsychosocial approach to treatment and psychological input seems a necessary adjunct to the medical interventions on offer. Unfortunately, the inclusion of psychological interventions in BPD treatment has been slow for various reasons, including psychologists' own historical reluctance to offer psychotherapy to this group of patients who were often perceived to be unable to benefit from such interventions (Fromm-Reichman, 1949).

This reluctance to offer psychosocial treatment to patients with BPD has dissipated somewhat in recent years and it is now much more common to see patients being offered Cognitive Behavioural Therapy (CBT) in particular, which is currently being evaluated by several research groups and is showing substantial promise (Michalak, Yatham and Lam, 2004). However, a typical course of CBT for BPD, with weekly sessions, lasts about six months in total and requires an advanced level of training which is unlikely to be found in an average multidisciplinary team (Scott and Todd, 2002). Thus it can be argued that the treatments being developed currently rely too heavily on staff time that is comparatively expensive, or of restricted availability, and that these treatments are therefore unlikely to be put into widespread practice in the publicly funded sector. From a public health standpoint it is therefore important to develop treatments that can be delivered by staff with relatively little training, using a limited number of sessions.

The present manual, setting out the Sorensen Therapy for Instability in Mood (STIM), is written for non-expert and expert clinicians alike and comprises a four-session (sixty-minute) intervention validated by research carried out at the University of Hertfordshire in 2003–4 (Sorensen, 2004; Sorensen, Done and Rhodes, submitted). The intervention is inspired by a number of publications including Bauer and McBride (1996), Miklowitz (2002) and Torrey and Knable (2002), but was developed from a theoretical or 'model-driven' perspective and builds on the theoretical writings of Ehlers, Frank and Kupfer (1988) and Goodwin and Jamison (1990) to construct a practical intervention with BPD. The intervention, which has proved highly successful for the clients taking part in the validating research (Sorensen, 2004; Sorensen, Done and Rhodes, submitted) on measures of hopelessness and perceived control over symptoms, was specifically written with the less experienced clinician in mind. It is hoped that, for instance, general practitioners, assistant and trainee psychologists under supervision, as well as more experienced mental health workers, will find it a useful instrument when working with the bipolar disordered client group.

The structure of the manual

Hopelessness is a key predictor of suicidal behaviour, which is well-established to be a serious problem in BPD (Beck, Weissman, Lester and Trexler, 1974; Goodwin and Jamison, 1990). Furthermore, hopelessness is likely to come about through the experience, central to the nature of BPD, of having no control over symptoms that repeatedly occur and wreck daily life. Hopelessness is thus linked to a lack of belief in one's future ability to control the various symptoms occurring and to the expectation that these symptoms will make life very difficult or 'hopeless'. The empirical data collected on learned helplessness (Seligman, 1974; 1975) show that this state of mind causes passivity and prevents the individual from discovering that conditions may have changed, so that the perceived helplessness is just and only that: perceived (Ibid.). Similarly for hopelessness, and in terms of treatment, an intervention that can increase the perceived control over symptoms is also likely to prompt renewed activity and actual attempts to control the unwanted states or symptoms. When this happens, it is important that clients have access to coping strategies that can disconfirm the perceived reasons to experience hopelessness which, according to basic behavioural principles, will otherwise be reinforced and become even more entrenched. It is therefore important that clients are given an empowering and non-deterministic understanding of the nature of BPD relapse (this happens in session one of the current treatment) before developing the actual coping strategies (which takes place in sessions two and three). Further, in order for the treatment to be consolidated and have long-term effects, the social network, which will often have experienced many, seemingly unpredictable, relapses, must also be moved to not reinforce or recreate the learned helplessness and hopelessness. This can be a challenging aspect of any therapeutic effort because people close to individuals with BPD may, themselves, have internalised a degree of helplessness and hopelessness as a result of seeing past relapses occur outside of the client's or their control. (Network inclusion skills are developed in session four.) As such, the structure of the STIM follows from the fact that an 'empowering' form of psycho-education in relation to BPD is, typically, necessary in order for a client to be open to learn relapse prevention and coping strategies. Such strategies are less likely to survive over time if the social network is not included in the reinforcement of a new belief system which states that (at least some) control over symptoms can be achieved.

Another key feature of the STIM is the development of an individualised handbook or workbook for the enhancement of coping. This handbook is developed as an integral and progressive part of the intervention. Clients are encouraged to develop and improve on the strategies and information contained in the handbook after the treatment has formally ended. It is hoped that the handbook will become a working document for the client and that this will give him or her a sense of taking more control over the illness than was previously possible.

Who can conduct the treatment?

Although the treatment is developed with the stated aim of providing the less experienced health worker with an easy-to-use treatment package, and while the treatment is not designed to delve deeply into psychological problems, it is important to understand that BPD is a serious mental disorder that often has consequences such as suicidal behaviours attached to it. As a result, it is up to the clinician responsible for the implementation of the treatment to ensure that adequate and appropriate supervision by an experienced and suitably qualified mental health worker is available before embarking on the intervention.

Independently of the therapist's level of expertise, the intervention should be conducted in the spirit of collaboration and with a high degree of shared responsibility for the progression of treatment between client and therapist. In relation to this the following techniques and approaches to therapy should be borne in mind as guiding principles with regard to the atmosphere and general style of the intervention:

- *Express empathy.* Listen to the client without criticism, judgement or blame. Do your best to listen reflectively and gain a clear understanding of the client's perspective and situation.
- *Do not argue.* Argumentation is not productive. Challenges to beliefs are best received if they are made with a genuinely open mind and in the spirit of exploration of different ways to look at a given issue.
- *Encourage self-efficacy.* The client is likely to need support and affirmation regarding beliefs related to the ability to change and control instability of mood. A word of caution: be *realistic*; BPD is typically a relapsing disorder and clients are not going to have all their problems solved by any one intervention.
- *Use open-ended questions.* During the discussion sections of the intervention use follow-up questions that cannot easily be answered with a categorical answer (such as 'Yes' or 'No'). This allows the client to engage and think more seriously about the issues.

Using this manual according to your needs and expertise

The conversational style in this manual may seem too prescriptive to the experienced mental health clinician who can stamp his or her own authority on the precise implementation and wording of the intervention. However, the style of writing is a deliberate attempt to make the therapy accessible to assistant psychologists, trainee psychologists, general practitioners, mental health nurses, etc. who often do much of the day-to-day work with bipolar disordered clients, but who do not necessarily feel confident in taking much control over how a therapy is conducted. As a result, and while this is not advisable, the manual is written in a style that, in theory, would allow a less experienced clinician to simply read it out, word for word, with a client.

The manual is written with individual therapy in mind, but it would be a relatively simple matter to change to a group format and in the process reach more clients while allowing the group participants to inspire and learn from each other during therapy. If the intervention is adapted to a group format it is suggested that session two and session three are extended to 120 minutes, or that two extra sessions be added to the standard structure of four sixty-minute sessions given in this manual.

Session 1

Information for the therapist

This session is designed to give clients an empowering and non-deterministic understanding of the nature of BPD relapse and to familiarise him or her with the collaborative therapeutic relationship promoted in this treatment. This is done via a description of BPD within a stress-vulnerability framework such as that developed by Zubin and Spring (1977), and the session should emphasise the client's ability to play an active part in managing the disorder and its related problems.

For the therapist it is vital to realise that this first session should set up the following sessions, in the sense that hope of a realistic nature regarding an increased degree of control over internal states should be instilled. This is a necessary first step in the treatment process, as many clients will come to treatment with past experiences indicating that no such control is possible. The first session should answer the question: "Why should I attempt to learn new behaviours and strategies?" while also providing general information about the disorder.

Welcome and short statement about the purpose of the treatment

Welcome and thank you for coming. The plan for what we will be doing over the next four sessions includes the development of both your knowledge and your coping strategies in relation to BPD, which you may know under its older name 'manic depressive illness'. During the four sessions we will look at what BPD is in general terms. We will look at what your particular BPD looks and feels like. We will discuss and describe the signs and symptoms of your depressions and manic episodes. We will look in detail at what can trigger them, which will then be related to what might be effective ways for you to be coping and living with BPD. At the end of the sessions you will leave here with a personal handbook for understanding and coping with the problems you encounter in relation to BPD. This handbook is made up from the worksheets that we will be using in the sessions and will be developed specifically in relation to your particular and individual experiences and needs. The hope is that you will then continue to update and improve on the handbook once the sessions have ended, so that you are always improving your ability to understand and cope with the disorder.

Guidelines for the intervention

A   While you have the right to stop participation at any time, it is important that you come to all sessions, as you, and we, will not be able to assess the benefits of the treatment until all the sessions have been completed.

B   My job is to help you plan a way to cope with difficulties, so if anything goes wrong or you have concerns, please let me know before you leave for the day so we can attempt to deal with them in the appropriate way.

C   [Give any service-specific guidelines regarding confidentiality, etc.]

Discussion

Do you have any comments or questions in relation to these guidelines? Do you have any thoughts on further guidelines or rules for the sessions that you would like to include or discuss?

Agenda and aims for session one

My goal for today is to cover and discuss:

1   What causes and influences BPD.
2   The so-called bipolar spectrum, which is everything from the average person's mood swings to full BPD.
3   Discrimination and stigma because of the diagnosis.
4   The outline of what we are doing next time.

It is also the first chance for us to get to know each other as we go along.

1. Client is educated about the spectrum of mood states and the patterns of the disorder (from normal mood fluctuations to BPD 1 and 2)

You are here today because, at some point, you have been given a diagnosis of BPD. But the disorder can express itself quite differently from person to person; it is important for you to understand the different ways that BPD can look for different people and also how it is related to so-called normal experiences that can have many of the same features. [Show and explain Figure 1 and point to worksheet 1 in the handbook.]

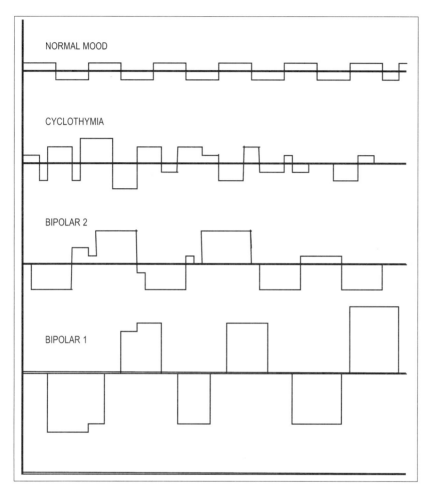

Figure 1 *Spectrum of mood states*

Figure 1 explained

The main features of BPD are basically exaggerated versions of normal mood swings and appear in all degrees of severity, for example, cyclothymic disorder, which consists of mood swings as seen in BPD, but not to the same degree.

In bipolar type 1 the mania is more extreme than in bipolar type 2, where it is called hypomania, which means 'mild mania'.

From the patterns in Figure 1 it is also clear that BPD is often, and typically, a relapsing disorder with episodes of mood fluctuations that can be more or less severe. So there are usually substantial periods with no signs of the disorder; this is similar to the way people can live with (say) diabetes, without symptoms of the illness constantly reminding them that they have it. This basically means that the disorder is under control. In diabetes you might be very careful about your diet, or you could be taking insulin regularly, or more likely you would be doing both. Similarly for BPD you can watch out for unhelpful or exaggerated stress, you can take the prescribed medication, or, as is most beneficial for most people, you can do both.

If a diabetic drinks a coke with a lot of sugar in, or forgets to take his or her insulin, then there will be a relapse and he or she will experience symptoms of diabetes. Similarly, someone with BPD who experiences excessive and unhelpful stress or stops his or her medication is likely to get symptoms of the disorder, i.e. to relapse.

Discussion

Can you relate the patterns in Figure 1 to your own experiences? Do you agree that BPD represents something normal that is being exaggerated? If so, what is being exaggerated?

The moods swings, whether they are up or down, can lead to an altered sense of reality. This is sometimes experienced as what professionals call psychosis; others have preferred to refer to the experiences as being spiritual in nature. There may be hallucinations, in the form of sensing something that others cannot agree is there. This often takes the form of seeing or hearing things which others cannot see or hear. Or you could have delusions, which are unusual beliefs. A typical example of a delusion is to believe that special messages are being delivered to you. But delusions can take many other forms and it is also common to experience extreme suspiciousness or paranoia. These experiences can be both frightening and confusing. However, in some cases people also report that they can have a pleasant content, and therefore function as a comfort in an otherwise confusing time.

Discussion

What sort of experiences have you had in relation to bipolar episodes? Have they only been unpleasant, or are there pleasant aspects to them for you?

We have now talked about the main features of the illness and we have discussed some typical experiences that can go with BPD. I have summarised this information in a worksheet, which also has a few more descriptive words about BPD. I suggest that we have a look at this worksheet now and you can tell me if there is anything that I have missed out or anything that I should not have included in the descriptions. [Go to worksheet 3 and explain to/discuss with client.]

2. Client is educated about the high prevalence of BPD and a discussion about stigma facilitates the therapeutic relationship

BPD affects about one in every hundred people over their lifetime; this is about the same as the number of people affected by diabetes. It does not discriminate between genders and it affects people from all walks of life; several famous and highly successful people have had the disorder. However, despite the fact that it is a relatively common occurrence, it is rarely discussed openly in the way that something like diabetes is. This can mean that people who have this type of problem can feel lonely and on their own with the problems that the disorder can cause. The reasons why people do not like to talk about having the disorder vary from person to person, but it is common to fear the stigma of being labelled, or to fear discrimination because of the diagnosis.

However, it is important to know that lots of people have it and that a likely reason why you probably do not know many people with the diagnosis (except in any patient groups that you attend) is that most do not discuss the illness openly outside the family or other very close relationships. It is also important to realise that many people manage the illness well and have fulfilled lives while living with the disorder.

Discussion

Do you know anyone with BPD? How is their life? Have you been discriminated against because of the disorder? Do you think that it is a good idea to be open about having the diagnosis? Are there situations where you would not tell people and situations where you always would?

3. A multi-model intervention strategy is argued for by presenting causes and influences within the stress-vulnerability model

Questions that many people with the diagnosis have are: "Why me?" and "What can cause an episode of illness?" In this treatment I differentiate between factors that caused the original onset of the disorder, and factors that influence how the disorder manifests itself later on. The reason for this is that these factors are not always the same.

Genetic factors are thought to play an important role in causing the initial episode of the disorder. Therefore having BPD or even depression in the family appears to make it more likely that someone would develop BPD themselves.

It is a little different when we look at subsequent episodes taking place after the initial one, because these so-called relapses into mania or depression look to be heavily influenced by other factors such as stress, sleep disruption, substance abuse, not taking medication, etc. These are all things that we can work at changing if we choose to do so, just like someone with diabetes can change what they eat or whether they take insulin.

Looking at the issues in this way means that BPD is not just a matter of psychological problems, or just a matter of a chemical imbalance in the brain. In fact it can be both of those things at the same time.

This means that a useful model for helping us to understand relapse in BPD has to take both of these aspects into account and combine them in a sensible manner. In other words, it makes sense to look at the disorder as an interaction between *biological factors*, such as reduction in the effects of chemicals in the brain, *psychological factors*, such as hopes, expectations, predictions and interpretations about things in your life, and *stress factors*, such as having a child that does not sleep through the night, conflict with a partner, a difficult job situation, moving house, financial difficulties, etc.

So we will all have a certain degree of vulnerability to bipolar episodes at the biochemical level and you may have been born with a tendency for over- or underproduction of certain chemicals that work in the brain to keep mood in a stable state [note to therapist: if client asks for details, this can be a number of chemicals yet unknown but norepinephrine, dopamine and serotonin are good candidates], or the nerve cells in your brain may not be using the chemicals in the best way possible.

Much of the time these vulnerabilities will not be having an impact on your day-to-day life. But when you encounter a lot of stress and this gets above a certain threshold, then the vulnerabilities can be expressed as depression or mania. So the biological vulnerability can impact on your psychological and emotional reactions to the stressful things going on in your life at that particular time. If we take away the stress that triggered the episode, then it is more likely that the biological vulnerability will no longer be expressed and a new depression or manic episode will be less likely to take place. We can learn from what has triggered episodes in the past, and thereby start to build up knowledge about the things that stress you in a way that should be avoided because they make it more likely that you will become ill.

Another way of looking at the same relationship between vulnerability and stress is to say that we have to balance our *basic vulnerability* and the *stress* we experience, with *protective strategies* that can help us reduce the stress levels and which will allow us to cope better with what life throws at us. [Discuss Figure 2 and point to worksheet 2.]

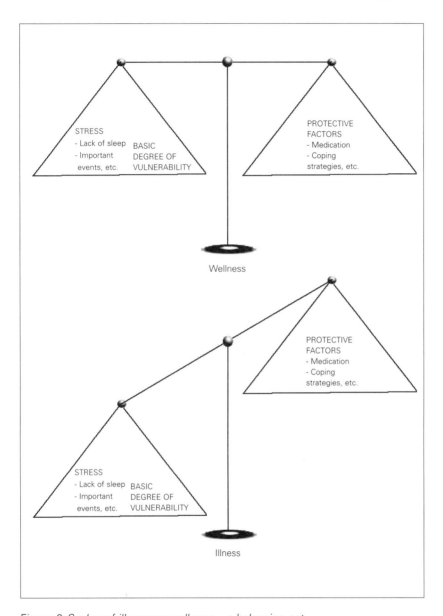

Figure 2 *Scales of illness or wellness – a balancing act*

Figure 2 explained

This model shows how someone with a high degree of genetic vulnerability, for example, if BPD has run in the family for several generations, would need a smaller amount of stress to see the scales tip in the direction of illness and an episode be triggered. Similarly, it shows that someone with very little genetic vulnerability would need to experience more stress to have an episode.

More important for what we are doing here, the model illustrates that there are things we can do to gain some control over the disorder. These are the 'protective factors' shown in the figure. If we get to know what particular stress factors to look out for, it becomes possible to shift the weight of the scales to a more balanced position by avoiding or managing the stress in question.

It follows from this that there are several different things we can do to reduce the risk of relapsing into illness, ranging from the way we work and live our lives generally, to the way we approach medication. These protective factors or strategies are some of the things that we will be looking at during the next sessions.

Discussion

Can you recognise the idea that stress makes it more likely that a relapse will take place? [Note to therapist: exams, job interviews, moving house, etc. are likely situations where relapses may have occurred in the past.] Have you experienced an episode coming out of the blue without any warning, if you look back to the time before the relapse?

Next session

Next time we will focus on the depressive side of BPD. You will develop the handbook with a list of your own first signs that indicate a relapse may be about to happen and you will develop your understanding of your individual symptoms and triggers for a depressive episode. The hope is that this will enhance your ability to manage the problems in a proactive way and therefore increase your ability to control the depressive side of the disorder.

So next time you will:

1 Develop a personal list of signs and symptoms of depression.
2 Develop a personal list of triggers for depression.
3 Develop a depression profile that is particular and individual to you (thoughts, behaviours and feelings characteristic of you when you are becoming depressed).
4 Determine personal criteria for when to react to changes in the depression profile and list the actions to take. ("When I feel and think in this way, I contact my GP", etc.)

Session 1
worksheet 1

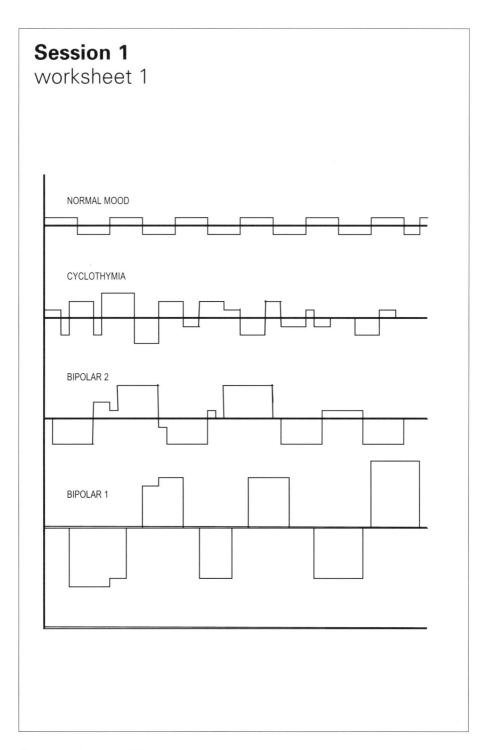

Spectrum of mood states

Session 1
worksheet 2

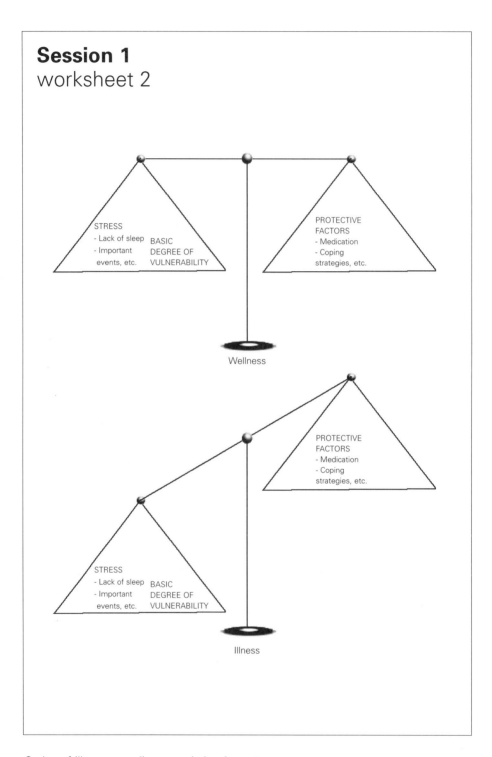

Scales of illness or wellness – a balancing act

Session 1
worksheet 3

The typical bipolar experience in brief

Mania

Emotions: Exaggerated and extreme happiness without relation to the realities of the particular situation. Alternatively, one can be very irritable or moods may shift rapidly and without obvious reason. Sometimes enhancement of one's senses takes place; this can be seen in increased colour perception or sharper hearing.

Thinking: It is typically difficult to concentrate, as one is easily distracted by many thoughts occurring at once. The thoughts can be accelerated, as can speech. It is not uncommon that the many thoughts are expressed in enhanced creativity.

Self-esteem: Inhibitions are decreased as one's importance in the world is perceived to be greater and therefore less determined by others' opinions. It is also common to experience paranoia, sometimes in the form of believing that others are out to get you because they are envious of your greater abilities.

Behaviour: Physical activity is typically increased substantially as a decreased need for sleep occurs. This activity can involve spending sprees, increased sexual activity (sometimes of a risky or personally atypical nature), increase in alcohol and/or drug use and a general tendency to get involved in risky behaviours and activities.

Depression

Emotions: Depressed, down, hopeless. In general terms a person in this state feels that all joy and pleasure in life has left him or her and will often not be easily convinced that such experiences will ever return.

Thinking:	Concentration, planning, memory and thought-functions in general are impaired and slowed down. It is not uncommon to have many thoughts about death and suicide.
Self-esteem:	Very hard on oneself, which can include actual self-hate based on a feeling of worthlessness.
Behaviour:	Reduced activity, extreme tiredness and lack of motivation. Sleep patterns are often disturbed, adding to the tiredness and lack of energy which is characteristic of depression.

Mixed states

In a mixed state any of the above experiences may be happening at the same time and it is possible to be full of energy (restlessness) while feeling very low in mood. Equally, one can be drained of thoughts and motivation to do anything while experiencing great restlessness and anxious energy.

Session 2

This session is designed to aid the client's awareness of his or her own early signs, symptoms and triggers for a depressive episode. This will enhance the ability to manage the disorder in a proactive and functional manner that is personally meaningful to the individual.

Agenda and aims for session two

1   Develop a list of signs and symptoms of depression individual to the client.
2   Develop a list of triggers for depression individual to the client.
3   Develop an individual depression profile (thoughts, behaviours and feelings characteristic of the individual client's depressive episodes).
4   Determine personal criteria for when to react to changes in the depression profile and list the actions to take.

Introduction to today's session

We saw last time that BPD is characterised by extreme mood swings that involve quite extensive changes in emotions, thinking and behaviour. Understanding how one's own particular illness expresses itself includes being able to recognise the symptoms that form a typical but individual pattern, and is a first step towards developing coping strategies that can eliminate, or at least limit, illness episodes recurring. This is very important because even the perfect plan for how to cope and what to do is not very useful if we do not know when to put the plan into action. Today we will develop your personal lists of signs, symptoms and triggers of depression. This will then lead us on to finding and describing your individual and unique depression profile made up of the thoughts, behaviours and feelings that go with your particular depression. This, in turn, will enable us to develop better criteria for when to react to changes in the depression profile, and we can then list the actions to take in order to combat the depression. Next week we will be doing something very similar with mania.

1. The development of a personal list of signs and symptoms of depression and the development of an individual depression profile

Thinking back to our last session and the worksheets you were given, we saw that depression is largely made up of the way a person thinks, feels and behaves. So while we know that certain symptoms must be present for a diagnosis of depression to be made, the experience of depression can reasonably be summed up by the particular thoughts, feelings and behaviours that characterise the individual depression, which will vary somewhat from person to person.

Discussion

Thinking back to our last session, what kind of experiences will a person have when he or she is depressed? [Note to therapist: if no examples are generated ask specifically about thoughts, feelings and actions/behaviours.] Does this general pattern correspond to your particular experiences with depression or do you think that your depressions are different in any way?

[Note to therapist: therapist writes down suggestions on board under the headings of Thoughts, Feelings and Behaviours. If the client does not generate sufficient examples the therapist suggests common symptoms and carefully checks that these are part of the client's experience of depression before including them on the list (see Appendix A for inspiration with regard to common symptoms). When a reasonable list has been generated, the therapist directs the client's attention to session two worksheet 1, Individual depression profile, and asks the client to check off symptoms that represent his or her particular depression and to add relevant symptoms not listed in the blank spaces, while checking off the first occurring warning signs of relapse with an F.]

Some of the symptoms you have listed are the same for every person with depression, but it is also important to note that your personal list is a 'cluster' of signs and symptoms that is personal to you; you might have signs or symptoms that someone else with the same diagnosis of depression would never experience as part of their individual depression profile.

In the same vein, the symptoms of depression can return in several different ways. They can come to you slowly and gradually, increasing in intensity and severity over time or sometimes they can develop quite quickly. Also, it is important to be aware that it is possible to be in the somewhat confusing situation of having both manic and depressed symptoms intermixed, as noted in worksheet 3 from session one.

Discussion

How have you experienced the occurrence or return of depression in the past?

2. The development of a personal list of triggers for relapse into depression

Last time I compared BPD to diabetes where sugar levels can go too high or too low because the body cannot regulate them in the appropriate way. In BPD it is mood that is not being regulated properly. If it goes too high you experience mania, too low and you experience depression. Both these phases of the illness will usually have some periods in between when you feel an average degree of stability in mood and therefore feel fine. However, it is the nature of BPD for depression or mania to return and, in a sense, it is part of the disorder to experience fluctuations in mood. You could say that mood instability is a characteristic of the disorder and stress can increase this instability.

Stress can be many things and not just negative things either. You can think of stress as the effect of good or bad life events – so anything that can stimulate your feelings or upset your pattern of daily life can be seen as stress. It is normal for us to respond to good and bad events happening to us with good and bad moods, but with BPD you may be more sensitive or vulnerable than most to the stresses of life. Furthermore, if stress triggers an illness episode, the episode can last long after the stress itself is gone. This makes the relation between the stress and the episode more difficult to see.

Discussion

What kind of stress do you think might bring on depression? If you think of your own episodes, can you recall if there was anything stressful going on just before you became depressed? What was it? Have you had any depressions where you could not see that there were any triggers?

[Therapist lists the examples of triggers provided by the client on the board and directs the client to session two worksheet 2, which is then completed.]

Now you have a list, or a *cluster*, of your personal signs and symptoms of depression that represents your individual depression profile. You also have a personal list of triggers or stressors that you have pinpointed as being involved in bringing about, or contributing to, the development of your depressive episodes.

3. Determine personal criteria for when to react to changes in the depression profile and list the actions to take

On worksheet 1 you have marked the first occurring warning signs of depression with an F. On worksheet 2 you have a list of potential triggers of depression based on what you know from the past. These lists are unlikely to be complete and you should always attempt to improve and expand on them even after this treatment has finished. Whenever you encounter any of the triggers or warning signs of depression that you have listed, you know that you should think about taking action so as not to become depressed. It is important that you read and learn your triggers and the first occurring warning signs well so that you are instantly aware when they occur. You should probably take out your handbook and have a look at them on a regular basis.

In worksheet 3, I have suggested some things that you can do to cope with depression in such situations. [Therapist reads through worksheet 3 with client. This includes going through worksheet 4.]

Discussion

If you look at items 7 and 8 on worksheet 3 you can see that they mention things to do and things not to do. From your experience, what are the things to do and not to do when at risk of becoming depressed? [Therapist writes own and client's suggestions on board and directs the client to write the examples in the space provided on the worksheet.]

Now if we look at worksheet 5 [therapist reads through worksheet 5 with client], you can see that there is room for the names and phone numbers of people you trust and think would be good to talk to in this type of situation. It is a good idea to put down more than one person in case you are unable to contact a particular person when the need arises. There is also room for you to add the phone numbers of your mental health worker or your GP. These could be important if you are at risk of becoming depressed. If you have these names and numbers ready please fill them in now. If not, please fill them in as soon as you get home today so as not to forget. You should also write in the most important things *to do* and *not to do*. Have a look at the lists we have done earlier today and write in what you feel is most important to you.

This little card is a very concise plan for what to do when at risk of becoming depressed. The card is designed to give you some simple, written information about what to do if you find yourself in a situation that might trigger a depressive episode. To have the information in written form can be very useful, even if you feel confident that you can easily remember these things, because memory and concentration are unlikely to be at their best when you are at risk of, or even just worried about, becoming depressed. Next time we will produce a similar card for mania and you will then be able to combine the two and have one card that can be carried with you, and that can guide you in what to do if at risk of becoming depressed or manic.

Next session

Next time we will focus on mania and we will do something very similar to what we have done today for depression, in the hope that this will help you manage and control the manic side of BPD in a proactive and adequate way that you can be happy with.

So next time you will:

1   Develop a personal list of signs and symptoms of mania.
2   Develop a personal list of triggers for mania.
3   Develop a mania profile that is particular and individual to you (thoughts, behaviours and feelings characteristic of you when you are becoming manic).
4   Determine personal criteria for when to react to changes in your mania profile and list the actions to take. ("When I feel and think in this way, I contact my GP", etc.)

Session 2
worksheet 1

Individual depression profile

Tick the symptoms you recognise from your own experience. Put an F by those that you feel are first indications that an episode might be under development.

Thoughts:

☐ Problems with doing your job or keeping a longer conversation going due to forgetting what is going on (i.e. losing track of what is being said).

☐ Concentrating is harder or takes up more energy than normal (i.e. it is difficult to know what is going on in a one-hour TV programme/film as you cannot keep your focus).

☐ Hallucinations or delusions (see worksheet 3 from session one).

☐ Persistent thoughts about other people being 'out to get you' or about them disliking you.

☐ Suicidal thoughts.

Add your own examples:

_____

_____

_____

_____

_____

_____

Feelings:

☐ Drained of energy.
☐ Feelings that you are useless to other people.
☐ Feeling low/down even when things that should have cheered you up occur.
☐ Easily angered and irritable (short fuse).
☐ Lack of self-confidence.
☐ Feeling guilty without knowing precisely why.
☐ Sadness all or most of the time.
☐ Appetite gone.

Add your own examples:

_____

_____

_____

_____

_____

_____

Behaviours:

☐ Eating too much or not enough.
☐ Sleeping too much or too little.
☐ Often tearful with no clear reason.
☐ Must be on the move at all times to combat restlessness.
☐ Stopping usual activities, being inactive.
☐ Seeking solitude/wanting to be alone.
☐ Difficulty starting or completing tasks.

Add your own examples:

_____

_____

_____

_____

_____

_____

Session 2
worksheet 2

Triggers of my depression

Put a mark in the boxes next to stress factors you believe have triggered depressive episodes for you in the past. Describe the triggers in the space provided and add any that are missing from the list (include any stress factor that you believe could trigger an episode even if this has not occurred to date).

☐ Negative events:

_____
_____
_____

☐ Positive events:

_____
_____
_____

☐ Stop or change to medication.
☐ Change in the use of substances (alcohol, cigarettes or drugs).
☐ Moving house.
☐ A major loss (job loss, death of a loved one, etc.):

_____
_____
_____

☐ Relationship breakdown.
☐ Conflicts with family, colleagues or others:

_____
_____
_____

☐ Working too hard.
☐ Partying too hard.
☐ Being on your own too much/feeling lonely.
☐ Not getting enough sleep.

Add your own examples:

_____
_____
_____
_____
_____
_____

Session 2
worksheet 3

Outline of strategies to combat depression

1 Contact your GP or mental health worker to 'touch base' and discuss the best way forward.
2 Check that you have taken your medication. If not, contact your GP or psychiatrist in charge of your medication.
3 Keep up your daily activities but do not go overboard and increase them dramatically.
4 Get your sleep! Good sleep habits should be put in place when you are feeling OK as changes can be difficult to make once depression has started (see worksheet 4).
5 Do not use alcohol or drugs. Whatever relief they give you will be short-lived and there is always a price to pay in relation to depression.
6 Be part of a support group and contact other members when needing to (go to the meetings even when you lack the motivation to do so).
7 Know what type of activity is right/meaningful for you and implement this.

See below for inspiration (A – N) with regard to things **to do** *and write them here:*

_____
_____
_____
_____
_____
_____

8 Know what is not helpful for you.

See below for inspiration (A – N) and write things **not to do** *here:*

_____
_____
_____
_____
_____
_____

A Phone a friend and tell them about your concerns.

B Do some relaxation.

C Do some exercise (run, walk, yoga, ride your bike, etc.).

D Do a hobby activity.

E Read a good book.

F Go shopping.

G Plan a day out for yourself and/or friends.

H Go and watch a movie (preferably a comedy).

I Talk to your mental health worker.

J Go and spend time with friends.

K Do not sit back and become passive.

L Tell yourself that "this will pass". Depressions only have a certain lifetime before they lift.

M Make sure you get some fresh air every day.

N Get up in the morning.

Session 2
worksheet 4

How to sleep well

1   Your bedroom should, if possible, be used only for sleeping. If you work, watch TV, eat, etc. in the bedroom, you will get used to being active where you want to sleep and this is counterproductive.
2   Sleep cannot be forced and sometimes it takes time. Relax.
3   Go to bed when you first begin to feel the need. Do not wait as you can start to 'wake up' and become less drowsy again.
4   Keep a routine for getting up and going to bed, and let this be the same on weekends as it is on weekdays. Our brain did not evolve to have a five-day week and does not like change in the sleep pattern from day to day!
5   Your body will allow only so much sleep in any twenty-four hour period. So, if you sleep or nap during the day, you will find it difficult to sleep at night.
6   Limit the night-time use of alcohol, tobacco and caffeine products to an absolute minimum.
7   Discuss the timing of medication intake with your doctor and let him or her know your concerns about sleep.
8   Exercise is tiring and will help you sleep but *not* if you do it immediately before going to bed.

Finally

Changes in sleep patterns take time and improvements may not be felt until two to three weeks after implementing the suggested habits and practices. Be patient; it will improve if you follow the above guidelines.

Session 2
worksheet 5

Plan for when at risk of becoming depressed

Plan for when at risk of becoming depressed

1   Have I taken my medication?
2   Am I overdoing the alcohol or am I using drugs?
3   What are the stress factors and triggers encountered and is there a simple way to change them?
4   Carry on with normal activities (i.e. go to work, social events, etc. as planned).
5   Most important things *to do:*

_____

_____

---

6   Most important things *not to do:*

_____

_____

7   Contact trusted person:
      Phone: _____
      Phone: _____
8   Contact GP or mental health worker:
      Phone: _____
      Phone: _____

This card can be cut out and carried with you. You may also want a copy in an accessible place at home.

Session 3

This session is designed to aid the client's awareness of his or her own early signs, symptoms and triggers for a manic episode. This will enhance the ability to manage the disorder in a proactive and functional manner that is personally meaningful to the individual.

Agenda and aims for session three

1 Develop a list of signs and symptoms of mania individual to the client.
2 Develop a list of triggers for mania individual to the client.
3 Develop an individual mania profile (thoughts, behaviours and feelings characteristic of the individual client's manic episodes).
4 Determine personal criteria for when to react to changes in the mania profile and list the actions to take.

Introduction to today's session

We saw in session one that BPD is typified by extremes in mood and we have talked about the related changes in thinking and behaviour that go with the disorder. In particular, last time we looked, in some detail, at the depressive side of the disorder and we discussed some strategies that can be used to manage the depression. We talked about how being able to recognise triggers, symptoms and especially the first signs that an episode of illness might be starting is a first step towards developing techniques or strategies that can prevent, or at least limit, a depressive episode. This same logic and approach is also true when looking at the manic side of BPD.

As a result, today we will be developing individual lists of signs, symptoms and triggers of manic episodes, specifically tailored to you and based on your past experiences of mania and on the things you believe could be helpful. This will allow us to develop an individual mania profile of thoughts, behaviours and feelings that go with your particular manic episodes. This, in turn, will enable us to develop better personal criteria for when to react to changes in the profile. We can then list the things to do in order to try to stop or reduce the impact of the manic episode. Remember that everything we develop here and include in the handbook should be seen as the beginning of an ongoing attempt to perfect the handbook and to help your general ability to cope with the mood swings encountered. As such the handbook can, and should, be updated and improved long after we have finished our sessions here.

1. The development of a personal list of signs and symptoms of mania and the development of an individual profile of mania

Thinking back to session one and the worksheets you were given then, it transpires that mania can largely be understood as being made up of the way a person thinks, feels and behaves. So, as was the case with depression, we know that in order for a diagnosis of mania to be made, particular criteria must be met, but that the experience of mania is basically about the way a person thinks, feels and behaves and this will vary from person to person.

Discussion

What is being manic like for you? [Note to therapist: it is often difficult (or embarrassing, so be sensitive) for a client to remember their manic episodes and it may be necessary to focus on what the client has been told by others.] Follow-up questions: Is it a positive/negative/neutral experience with regard to thoughts/emotions/behaviours?

[Therapist writes down client suggestions on board under the headings of Thoughts, Feelings and Behaviours. If the client does not generate sufficient examples the therapist suggests common symptoms and carefully checks that these are part of the client's experience of mania before including them on the list (see Appendix B for inspiration with regard to common symptoms). When a reasonable list has been generated, display and consider session three worksheet 1, Individual mania profile, and ask the client to check off symptoms that represent his or her particular experience of mania and to add relevant symptoms not listed in the blank spaces, while checking off the first occurring warning signs of relapse, using an F.]

What you have now is a list of symptoms and the first appearing signs of mania, which is individual and possibly unique to you. It is important to work on updating and reading the list often, so as to get to know it well. Knowing the list well is what will allow you to notice and recognise the first signs of a relapse into mania. It is what will make it possible for you to implement coping strategies that will eliminate or reduce the impact of the episode. The sooner you can start implementing the strategies used to control or limit mania, the better your chances of actually combating and controlling it are likely to be.

Manic signs and symptoms can return in several ways. They can come to you slowly and gradually, increasing in intensity over time or sometimes they return quite quickly. As mentioned in our last session, it is possible to have both manic and depressed symptoms at the same time and to see them increase in intensity simultaneously.

Discussion

What has the pattern been for you with regard to the development of mania? (Quick or slow development.)

2. The development of an individual list of triggers for relapse into mania

In this treatment we have compared BPD with diabetes where sugar levels can go too high or too low because the body cannot regulate them and we have discussed how in BPD it is the mood that is not being regulated properly and which can go too 'high' or too 'low'. We have also seen that stress can increase this instability.

As we saw in last week's session, stress can take many forms, both positive and negative in origin, and can be thought of as anything that takes up energy or stimulates feelings and upsets the basic routines of life. We looked at how someone with a basic vulnerability to BPD can be thought of as having a greater than average sensitivity to certain things occurring. We saw that if stress triggers an illness episode, the episode can last long after the stress itself is gone and after a while it can be difficult to identify the original trigger.

Discussion

What kind of stress do you think might bring on a manic episode? Do you have any experience of mania where you could not see what had triggered it? What has triggered mania for you? What do you think could trigger an episode in the future? [Therapist lists the examples of triggers provided by the client on the board and directs the client to worksheet 2 which is then completed.]

Now you have a list, or a *cluster*, of your personal signs and symptoms of mania that represents your individual mania profile. You also have a personal list of triggers or stressors that you have pinpointed as being involved in bringing about, or contributing to, the development of your manic episodes.

3. Determine personal criteria for when to react to changes in the individual mania profile and list the actions to take

On worksheet 1 you have marked the first occurring warning signs of mania with an F and on worksheet 2 you have a list of potential triggers of manic episodes based on what you know from the past. These lists are unlikely to be complete and you should always attempt to improve and expand on them and the handbook in general even after this treatment has finished. Whenever you encounter any of the triggers or warning signs of mania that you have now listed, you know that you should think about taking action so as not to become manic. It is important that you read and learn your triggers and the first occurring warning signs well so that you are instantly aware when they occur. You should probably take out your handbook and have a look at them on a regular basis. In worksheet 3, I have suggested some things that you can do to cope with mania. [Therapist reads through worksheet 3 with client.]

Discussion

If you look at items 7 and 8 on the worksheet you can see that they mention things to do and things not to do. From your experience, what are the things to do and not to do when at risk of becoming manic? [Therapist writes own and client's suggestions on board and directs the client to write the examples in the spaces provided on the worksheet.]

As we saw last time, part of good coping is good sleep habits, so just to make sure that it is clear how important this is, I've included worksheet 4 about good sleep habits again. This is equally important for depression and mania. [Worksheet 4 is considered.]

Now if we look at worksheet 5 [therapist reads through worksheet 5 with client] you can see that there is room for the names and phone numbers of people you trust and think would be good to talk to in this type of situation. It is a good idea to put down more than one person, as you may not be able to contact a particular person when the need arises. There is also room for you to add the phone numbers of your mental health worker or your GP. These could be important if you are at risk of becoming manic. If you have these names and numbers ready please fill them in now. If not, please fill them in as soon as you get home today, so as not to forget. You should also write in the most important things *to do* and *not to do*. Have a look at the lists we have done earlier today and write in what you feel is most important to you.

This little card is a very concise plan for what to do when at risk of becoming manic. The card is designed to give you some simple, written information about what to do and not to do if you find yourself at risk or in a situation that might trigger a manic episode. To have the information in written form can be very useful, even if you feel confident that you can easily remember these things, because memory and concentration are unlikely to be at their best when you are at risk of, or even just worried about, becoming manic.

This little card now contains the most important things to do when you notice the first signs of relapse or face triggers of mania and, with the information from the previous session on depression, you can now transfer all the information onto a combined card. [Note to therapist: give combined depression/mania card and ask client to transfer information from the two separate cards onto this.] This card gives you a super-brief summary of the essence of the handbook as it looks so far, that can be carried with you and can provide guidance whenever needed. Keep the card with you at all times and read it at regular intervals so that you know whether it needs to be updated or changed in any way. By reading it regularly you will also be more likely to consider it and use it when the need arises.

Next session

Next time we will look at how the developed strategies can fit into, and be strengthened by, the way you live your life in general, at home and at work. Because this is an important aspect of how you cope and feel about life in general we will look at how BPD might be experienced by the people around you. We will discuss if and what you should communicate to them about your situation and about BPD in particular. We will also look at some ways to think about and handle employment and employers in a way that minimises the stress you experience. [Note to therapist: if client is not in employment, refer to the possibility of future employment, volunteer work or any other activity that fills a substantial amount of time in the person's life.]

So next time we will:

1   Discuss information relating to BPD for family members. What should they know?
2   Look at common problems arising in the family and in the wider social network as a consequence of BPD. We will also look at how these can be handled and we will work on some communication techniques that can be helpful in this regard.
3   Finally, we will review the handbook and say goodbye. [Note to therapist: if a booster session is planned this will be set up for two to three months post treatment.]

Session 3
worksheet 1

Individual mania profile

Tick the symptoms you recognise from your own experience. Put an F by those that you feel are first indications that an episode might be under development.

Thoughts:

☐ Problems keeping a conversation/stream of thought due to loss of interest (i.e. losing track because you are thinking about the next topic).
☐ Concentrating is harder because your thoughts are racing ahead at great speed.
☐ Hallucinations or delusions (often about having special powers).
☐ Persistent thoughts about other people being 'out to get you' (paranoia).
☐ Your thoughts are experienced as being very clear.
☐ Self-obsession or thoughts centred on yourself much of the time.

Add your own examples:

_____

_____

_____

_____

_____

_____

Feelings:

☐ Full of energy.
☐ Feeling that you are superior to other people.
☐ Emotions change very quickly.
☐ Easily angered and irritable (short fuse).
☐ Increased self-confidence.
☐ Fooling that "the world is at my feet and nothing will ever go wrong for me".
☐ Very to extremely happy.

Add your own examples:

_____
_____
_____
_____
_____
_____

Behaviours:

☐ Engaging in more risky activity (dangerous driving, etc.).
☐ Sleeping little compared to usual need.
☐ Engaging in more sexual activity.
☐ Always on the move.
☐ Going out more (parties, nightclubs, etc.).
☐ Going on spending sprees.
☐ Starting many new projects or activities at once without finishing them.

Add your own examples:

_____
_____
_____
_____
_____
_____

Session 3
worksheet 2

Triggers of my mania

Put a mark in the boxes next to stress factors you believe have triggered manic episodes for you in the past. Describe the triggers in the space provided and add any that are missing from the list (include any stress factor that you believe could trigger an episode even if this has not occurred to date).

☐ Negative events:

_____

_____

_____

☐ Positive events:

_____

_____

_____

☐ Stop or change to medication.
☐ Change in the use of substances (alcohol, cigarettes or drugs).
☐ Moving house.
☐ A major loss (job loss, death of a loved one, etc.):

_____

_____

_____

☐ Relationship breakdown.
☐ Conflicts with family, colleagues or others:

_____

_____

_____

☐ Not getting enough sleep.
☐ Going on holiday or other drastic change in daily routine.
☐ Working too hard.

Add your own examples:

_____

_____

_____

_____

_____

_____

_____

Session 3
worksheet 3

Outline of strategies to combat mania

1 Contact your GP or mental health worker to 'touch base' and discuss the best way forward.
2 Check that you have taken your medication. If not, contact your GP or psychiatrist in charge of your medication.
3 Keep up your daily activities but do not go overboard and increase them dramatically.
4 Get your sleep! Good sleep habits should be put in place when you are feeling OK as changes can be difficult to make once mania has started (see worksheet 4).
5 Do not use alcohol or drugs; they are likely to make things worse.
6 Be part of a support group and contact other members when you need to (go to the meetings even when you lack the motivation to do so).
7 Know what type of activity is right/meaningful for you and implement this.

*See below for inspiration (A – L) with regard to things **to do** and write them here:*

_____
_____
_____
_____
_____
_____

8 Know what is not helpful for you.

*See below for inspiration (A – L) and write things **not to do** here:*

_____
_____
_____
_____
_____
_____

A   Phone a friend and tell them about your concerns.
B   Do some relaxation or yoga.
C   Do a quiet hobby activity.
D   Read a good book.
E   Take a long hot bath.
F   Talk to your mental health worker.
G   Go and spend time with one or two friends; stay away from crowds.
H   Do not put yourself in situations with a lot of stimuli (light, noise, etc.).
I   Hand over control of credit- and store-cards to a trusted person.
J   Arrange with employer to do less demanding work for a few days.
K   Write in your diary or write letters to friends (not to be overdone).
L   Do not make commitments to friends or others for a few days.

Session 3
worksheet 4

How to sleep well

1 Your bedroom should, if possible, be used only for sleeping. If you work, watch TV, eat, etc. in the bedroom, you will get used to being active where you want to sleep and this is counterproductive.
2 Sleep cannot be forced and sometimes it takes time. Relax.
3 Go to bed when you first begin to feel the need. Do not wait as you can start to 'wake up' and become less drowsy again.
4 Keep a routine for getting up and going to bed, and let this be the same on weekends as it is on weekdays. Our brain did not evolve to have a five-day week and does not like change in the sleep pattern from day to day!
5 Your body will allow only so much sleep in any twenty-four hour period. So, if you sleep or nap during the day, you will find it difficult to sleep at night.
6 Limit the night-time use of alcohol, tobacco and caffeine products to an absolute minimum.
7 Discuss the timing of medication intake with your doctor and let him or her know your concerns about sleep.
8 Exercise is tiring and will help you sleep but *not* if you do it immediately before going to bed.

Finally

Changes in sleep patterns take time and improvements may not be felt until two to three weeks after implementing the suggested habits and practices. Be patient; it will improve if you follow the above guidelines.

Session 3
worksheet 5

Plan for when at risk of becoming manic

Plan for when at risk of becoming manic
1   Have I taken my medication?
2   Am I overdoing the alcohol or am I using drugs?
3   What are the stress factors and triggers encountered and is there a simple way to change them?
4   Carry on with normal activities but do not overdo them.
5   Most important things *to do:*
    _____
    _____

6   Most important things *not to do:*
    _____
    _____

7   Contact trusted person:
    Phone: _____
    Phone: _____
8   Contact GP or mental health worker:
    Phone: _____
    Phone: _____

This card can be cut out and carried with you. You may also want a copy in an accessible place at home.

Session 3
worksheet 5a

Combined card (double-sided)
Concise plans for when at risk of becoming depressed or manic

Plan for when at risk of becoming depressed
1   Have I taken my medication?
2   Am I overdoing the alcohol or am I using drugs?
3   What are the stress factors and triggers encountered and is there a simple way to change them?
4   Carry on with normal activities (i.e. go to work, social events, etc. as planned).
5   Most important things *to do:*
    _____
    _____

6   Most important things *not to do:*
    _____
    _____

7   Contact trusted person:
    Phone: _____
    Phone: _____
8   Contact GP or mental health worker:
    Phone: _____
    Phone: _____

Plan for when at risk of becoming manic

1   Have I taken my medication?
2   Am I overdoing the alcohol or am I using drugs?
3   What are the stress factors and triggers encountered and is there a simple way to change them?
4   Carry on with normal activities but do not overdo them.
5   Most important things *to do:*

_____
_____

6   Most important things *not to do:*

_____
_____

7   Contact trusted person:
     Phone: _____
     Phone: _____
8   Contact GP or mental health worker:
     Phone: _____
     Phone: _____

This card can be cut out and carried with you. You may also want a copy in an accessible place at home.

Session 4

This session is designed to integrate all the illness management strategies developed in sessions two and three with the client's social and work-related activities. This includes education about how his or her family might experience BPD and will also develop communication skills and an individually tailored approach to employment and employers. [Note to therapist: if the client is not in employment, relate these aspects of the session to the possibility of future employment, volunteering activity or any other activity that takes up much of the client's time.]

Agenda and aims for session four

1 Gain insight into the importance of involving the client's family in coping.
2 Gain insight into adaptive communication skills regarding BPD.
3 Develop a plan for how to manage work situations, including communication with the client's employer.

Introduction to today's session

Following a depression or a manic episode you will most likely look forward to getting things back to 'normal' with your partner, your wider family and at work. It is however important to realise that the experiences of the illness, and of you as a person, may have changed the perception that people around you have of you.

People are often angry and can blame you for being ill, or they can be extremely worried that you may become ill again and will therefore treat you in what feels like an over-protective or even patronising manner. Your colleagues may not know how to handle the situation and can start distancing themselves from you as a result of fear or misunderstandings about what could cause a relapse. Equally, your employer may think that you are not up to the job and could start marginalising you in the workplace, passing you over for promotion, or start to neglect your professional development. So it is important to work out how to handle these situations and to make the necessary adjustments so that people can see you for who you are and so that you can be an effective person at home and at work.

These are the kind of questions we will be looking at today. If you are not currently working, the part of today's session dealing with work is still relevant to you, as you might take up employment in the future, or you can relate the discussion to other aspects of your life that may be stressful in the same way as employment can be stressful.

1. Family members and BPD: the need for good communication skills

Depression, and maybe in particular mania, involve some behaviour that can be very difficult to comprehend from the outside, and from the perspective of a family member an understandable reaction is frustration. For instance, this can take the form of confusion and annoyance: "But *why* could you not get out of bed and eat a little bit of breakfast?" or "But *why* did you go out and spend all our rent money on stuff that we don't really need?" It is common that people get frustrated, not only with you, but also with themselves because they care about you and feel that they should help but do not know how. When people are frustrated and perhaps feel some guilt that they are unable to help, they often turn to blaming you for the illness, or to being extremely vigilant with regard to any sign of the illness, which can lead you to feel that you are constantly being watched or treated like an irresponsible child.

Blaming can take several forms but will typically involve criticising you for not getting better, or for not trying hard enough to get and stay better. It can involve name-calling or references to you being a bad person, or it can involve accusations that you are selfish because you, for instance, enjoy being a little manic, etc.

Discussion

Have you ever felt blamed for being ill? If so, what happened? Do you understand why someone could blame you for the illness?

The possibility that some people are so worried about a relapse that they become over-vigilant with regard to looking for any signs of symptoms is clearly based on them caring for your well-being, but it can in fact be very stressful for you. This is because being worried can lead to an over-inclusiveness in thinking about the disorder amongst your loved ones, so that many of the normal things you do are seen as part of BPD when they are really not. For example, if you have had a bad day at work and feel a bit upset about this and your reactions are not taken for what they really are, 'normal', but are seen as a sign of relapse into depression, you are likely to feel misunderstood and maybe humiliated and this is in itself stressful.

Discussion

Have people around you been worried about relapse to the degree that they treated you differently or even made you feel that they thought you were a child? What happened?

The worst-case scenario is that over-inclusive thinking amongst people around you, with much of what you do or say being interpreted as signs that an episode of the illness is about to happen, could actually stress you to a degree that initiates a relapse. If, for example, you have a good day and feel happy without any particular or clear reason, your relatives could take this as a sign that you are becoming manic and ask you repeatedly whether you have taken your medication, or pressure you to go to see your mental health worker. This, in turn, could make you angry and irritable, i.e. "Why can I not just be happy without being seen as ill? And why do you nag me about this all the time?" Your relatives could then see this anger, or irritability, as proof that you are indeed becoming manic and they would then be even more inclined to ask questions about your medication and about whether you should go and see the mental health worker. In the end this could be a vicious circle that is very difficult to break and which continues to increase the tension and the stress put on you, possibly with mania as the final outcome, which, in turn, would confirm your relatives' beliefs, i.e. "Told you, we were right all along when we said that an episode was beginning to take form." This is obviously a negative outcome and could increase the likelihood that your relatives will react in a similar fashion next time they see you being happy, angry, sad, creative and so on without any obvious reasons. It is therefore very important that we find a way to break this vicious circle.

Discussion

Can you recognise this pattern? The worst possible outcome is that this type of pressure actually triggers an episode. Do you think that that has happened to you?

If you are experiencing one or more of the problems we have discussed so far today, the good news is that we will now look at how they can be addressed.

2. Techniques and strategies for educating the family and other important people

The first step is to realise that even if relatives or friends have made an effort to understand and listen to your explanations, have spoken to your GP and your mental health worker and have read up on BPD, they can still be unclear about what it really means to have the disorder and about what the future is likely to hold for you and them. It is very important that you take it upon yourself to educate close friends and relatives. It is a good idea to do this little by little when you think people are in a receptive mood and you should do this even if you do not perceive there to be any problems with the degree of understanding held by the people around you. This is because we don't know what the future will bring and it is better to be discussing these things when you don't have any problems, as these conversations can be more difficult during periods of high stress, such as when you are coming out of an episode of the illness. The issues should also be discussed following a relapse and during the recovery period. But these discussions will be much easier to have if they are simply repeating something that was already put on the agenda during a period when you were stable in mood and not directly affected by a relapse.

[Worksheet 1 is explained. It is suggested that participants photocopy and give worksheet 1 to relatives and other significant people in their lives, and that they make themselves available to answer any questions from significant others arising from the worksheet.]

It is important to develop a relaxed, but also precise, way of talking about the disorder with your family and other people who are close to you. Different ways of discussing what someone has experienced in relation to your symptoms and behaviours when ill can indicate differences in beliefs about what causes you to act in a certain way. For example, it is much easier for your partner or other family members to be understanding and supportive of you if they believe that your extreme impatience or angry outbursts are the results of an illness phase rather than the results of you changing into a grumpy or even aggressive person in general. Similarly, they should be helped to understand that the illness can put you in a depressed mood or make it difficult to concentrate on, and remember, what they are saying to you without you having become insensitive or permanently 'miserable' as a person.

Discussion

Do you feel that your relatives have an adequate understanding of BPD or do you need to educate them about it? [Note to therapist: if the client is a parent also, ask and discuss: Do you think that a special effort should be made to give your children an understanding of BPD? How should this be done? What are some good terms to use with children when describing what it is like to be depressed/manic?]

3. Communication skills

Ability to communicate in an effective way with the people around you is linked to good coping with BPD and with general well-being for you and them. The skills we will look at now are very important and you need to practise them on a regular basis, preferably when you are well, unstressed and feel stable in mood, as this makes them easier to use when you are ill and need them most.

4. Attentive engagement (AE)

When you are under a lot of stress or pressure, such as that caused by episodes of illness, you will most likely find it difficult to pay attention to the problems of others, even when they are reported by people who are important to you, such as family members or close friends. However, when you feel stressed it is also likely that the important people in your life experience some of this stress and that they feel a need for your support. If you are perceived to be unwilling to give this support, to at least some degree, it then becomes more likely that the people you rely on for support will find it harder and less appealing to do some of the things that interfere with their life, but which will aid your recovery. For example, they might not refrain from putting you under pressure to go to a concert or a movie that they have been looking forward to, but which could be over-stimulating for you if you are experiencing some of the first signs of a potential manic state.

In other words, they might 'force' their needs through if you are not seen to be responding and paying attention to the needs that they are expressing. Similarly, they are more likely to criticise you in a manner that can be stressful to you if they do not feel that you are taking adequate account of their concerns, wants and needs.

This illustrates why it is important for your illness management to help your relatives handle their anger or frustration by listening and explicitly showing an understanding of their point of view. When coming out of an episode of the illness, or when feeling under pressure generally, this can sound like a very daunting task, but much can be achieved by relatively simple and fairly undemanding means. This is because your relatives and friends, most likely, are looking for understanding and a reasonable level of attention to their needs, rather than for you to solve their problems or for you to be very active in what you do together. Therefore, what is required is an attentive engagement with what is going on for the people around you. This requires you to take time to listen and to make sure you fully understand what is going on, while also showing that you are making this effort. In the past much attention has been given to what has been called 'active or reflective listening' which can be useful techniques for showing that you care about what a speaker is saying. You can obtain good reading material on this if you are interested in learning more. [Note to therapist: if the client wants more information on active listening techniques give relevant references, such as Miklowitz and Goldstein (1997).] However, in this programme what is called attentive engagement (AE) broadens the definition of good communication from the focus on listening, and AE stresses that the context and the whole set of communication tools at our disposal are important (including body language and how we place ourselves in relation to the person we are attending to). [Go through worksheet 2 with client.]

Discussion

Do you have any questions or comments about AE?

In AE the focus is very much on the needs and feelings of the people who are important to you but this does not mean that you, at other times, should not ask for help or make sure that they understand how their behaviour can be more or less helpful to your coping. However, some of the principles from AE also apply when you want people to listen to you. For instance, if you want someone to change their behaviour in any way, it is important that you first think about what the situation would look like from their perspective and that you are willing to listen to their perspective. This attitude will make it more likely that they will listen to you and will improve the chance that they will be willing to change the behaviour in question. It is also very important that you focus on your goal rather than on what you feel is wrong with a given behaviour. In fact, if you criticise someone they are often more likely to continue the criticised behaviour than if you had said nothing at all!

Discussion

Do you agree that change seldom comes as a result of criticism? How do you react if people criticise you? Do you tend to change the criticised behaviour?

The alternative to criticising is to ask for change by informing someone what you would like to see. This is much more effective as it makes it clear what you would like to see without making a problem out of what is going on at present.

To illustrate this point, I wonder which of these statements, designed to change someone's tendency to be over-inclusive with regard to when BPD is relevant, do you think is more likely to get the desired result [therapist reads out the following]: "I'm really fed up that we can't have a simple conversation about my future without you bringing up my illness!" or "It's very important to me that I can talk about and plan my future like any other person. After all, we could all get ill."

Discussion

Which one of these statements do you think is most likely to get the desired result? Why? [Note to therapist: stating something in a positive manner makes it much easier to accept.]

This type of positive communication is a skill that needs to be practised, but you will find that the more you practise the more natural it becomes. This is something that you should be aiming for, because if it is not part of your normal way of speaking, then it is unlikely to happen when you are under pressure and need it the most. So again, the lesson is to practise when you are feeling good and when there is no tension in the air. It might feel a bit artificial at first, but this will soon pass, once you feel the benefits of this type of communication.

Discussion

Can you recognise from relationships with family members or friends that criticising is often met with defensiveness? Would it be a good idea to involve your family or friends in practising the more positive types of communication?

5. Managing BPD at work

When discussing how to be successful at work it is obviously very important to work at maintaining a stable mood in order to offer an employer what they are looking for, i.e. effective and reliable employees. This can be seen as another good reason to take medication on a regular basis. However, it is also essential to realise that the degree of support within the work environment, and the manner in which you approach work and the workplace itself, are important factors in relation to your stability of mood. The key issues then become how you manage to find the right balance between having an interesting job that challenges you in the way you want it to, and keeping work hours, general stimulation and stress levels at a level that does not, directly or indirectly, cause an illness episode to happen or become worse.

Discussion

Do you think that having BPD affects your employment? In what way has that happened? Some people report that BPD, and in particular the milder states of mania, can enhance their job performance. Do you recognise this from your own life? If so, are there any dangers in 'using' mania in this way?

A situation where it is often a good idea to be extra vigilant about a possible relapse is when you start a new job or return to your job after an illness episode. In this situation we often want to impress our employers, and show them that we can offer the company something important despite having BPD. This can result in a feeling of needing to over-achieve at work, sometimes even to a degree where you might feel 'driven' or compulsive about your work. This can, in turn, lead you to feeling down and tired at the end of the working day, and can also result in disturbed sleep patterns, with little sleep during the week and then many hours of sleep at the weekend. It is as if the pattern of BPD moves into the way you structure your work and home life, with hypomania being present at work and depression being present at home.

One of the things worth thinking about with regard to work is that research has shown that situations involving reward that promises more, such as a promotion, that can motivate and increase your drive towards other goals (Lam et al., 2003; Johnson et al., 2000 [give specific references if interested]), can trigger mania. The logical conclusion from this is that you *can* have a fulfilling work life, but it needs to be managed.

Discussion

What are the things that need managing for you when looking at work and the ability to maintain stability of mood?

Some of the things that often need to be considered are:

- The job itself (what are you doing and could/should this be done differently?).
- The work setting.
- Your employer (he or she can also play an important part in maintaining wellness).

To help avoid the stress and trigger factors that we have discussed during the last few sessions you should think carefully before taking up any job that includes shifting patterns (such as day work one week and night-time work the next); jobs with a lot of sudden/unscheduled social stimulation and demands for socialisation; jobs with little 'off-time' or which include a permanent on-call element; jobs with frequent travel across time zones or a lot of interpersonal stress. This does not mean that you cannot work in an environment where these stress factors exist, just that they need to be managed extra carefully and that some arrangement may need to be negotiated with your employer.

In order to come to an agreement with your employer, you first need to make sure that they know that you have BPD.

Discussion

Can you give me some reasons why not to tell your employer about your condition? Can you give me some reasons why it would be a good idea to tell your employer? Could you use worksheet 1 to tell your employer about BPD? [Worksheet 3 is completed and the client is asked if and when they are going to approach their employer.]

End of treatment

Over the last few weeks you have developed an individualised plan for coping with the particular BPD that you live with. This all adds up to an individual handbook for how to deal with difficult issues such as situations where you notice triggers of a relapse into illness, or where you spot the first signs that an episode of depression or mania might be happening. You have a super-concise version of what to do in such situations on a card that you can carry with you everywhere. You have also looked at some of the difficulties that may arise in family and work aspects of life, and have material to share with family members in order to educate them about the disorder and about the things that you might find challenging. This includes some strategies to improve the way you speak to the people close to you about the disorder. You have also now developed a plan for the things you would like to see improved at work, or, alternatively, a list of things that you will think about if you were to take up employment in the future.

Remember that many of the skills we have talked about are things that benefit from practice, so read your handbook often and try to the best of your ability to implement the things that you have decided would benefit you. Practice makes perfect, so do not despair if you do not get everything right the first time. No one does.

Are there any questions before we look through the handbook and remind ourselves what is included? [Note to therapist: if a booster session is planned this will be set up for two to three months post treatment.]

[Note to therapist: go through handbook and address any problems in understanding, while emphasising that the handbook should be updated and improved on by the client following treatment and as he or she thinks of more things to include.]

Session 4
worksheet 1

Brief fact sheet on bipolar disorder (BPD) for family and friends

What does it mean to have BPD?

BPD was previously called manic depressive illness and is a medical diagnosis used to describe people who are prone to drastic mood swings. In most cases this will involve going from being very energetic or 'high' (manic) for periods of time, to being almost entirely without energy and very 'low' (depressed) for, typically, somewhat longer periods of time (weeks to several months is not unusual in depression). About one in every hundred people has BPD, which is about the same number of people with diabetes. So it is a fairly common illness.

What causes BPD?

BPD is thought to be related to having an imbalance of chemicals in the brain and to the way that brain cells communicate with each other using these chemicals. Having BPD is in no way a choice and it is possible that an individual with the illness has inherited the tendency for the disorder from blood relatives, as genetics appear to play an important part in why people develop the disorder. The mood swings that a person with BPD experiences are also affected by stress and the things experienced in life more generally, such as sudden changes, being overworked, lack of sleep or other forms of stress.

How does one recognise BPD in a person?

What you, as a friend or a relative, may see in a person with this disorder can be varied. It is likely that he or she, when experiencing mania, will feel extremely happy and excited without any clear reasons for these emotions, or he or she may feel very differently and be easily angered and very irritable, again without there being any obvious reason for these emotions. The person's thoughts about him- or herself and the world will also most likely be altered when manic and he or she could, for instance, believe that 'someone is out to get me' when, in fact, they are not. The person with

BPD can also have grandiose thoughts about being able to do rather fantastic things and think that he or she is the only person in the world who is able to do these things.

The thoughts a person has during mania can be very fast and will often be experienced as if they are running out of control, so it is common for a person in a manic state to be rather impulsive in matters of money and other aspects of life. Similarly, the person experiencing mania will also be easy to distract from what he or she is doing at any one time. Further, mania means that a person is likely to talk faster, sleep much less and to express many ideas, some of which will not be realistic.

During periods where a bipolar person feels depressed and low, it is possible to see some of the symptoms mentioned before under mania, such as feeling irritable and having difficulty concentrating. But the main features of the low periods are typically feeling down, slow, sad, bad, guilty, fatigued and sometimes anxious. Also, the bipolar individual may lose interest in things or people that he or she otherwise cares for, and may experience sleep problems in the form of sleeping too much or finding it difficult to get to sleep at night. Similarly, eating can be difficult because loss of appetite may occur or you may see a tendency towards eating too much ('comfort eating').

A person in such a state of mind may contemplate suicide or actually attempt to take his or her own life, which illustrates that BPD is something that needs to be managed well, as the suicidal thoughts will most often be related to being in an episode of the illness and not a reflection on how the person feels about life when not depressed or manic.

Finally, it should be noted that it is possible to have the bipolar diagnosis without experiencing depression, as the defining feature of the diagnosis is mania.

Treatment

Treatment most likely includes one of a range of mood-stabilising drugs prescribed by a psychiatrist and may also involve taking anti-depressants in order to help control both depression and any anxiety symptoms that form part of the individual illness profile.

It can also be useful for a person with BPD, and for people close to him or her, to go to a talking therapy, be it family therapy or another form of counselling. Likewise, it can be helpful to belong to a support group of people who understand BPD from personal experience and who can therefore share their knowledge about issues to do with stress management, communication skills, effects and side-effects of medication, hints about how to obtain the best possible treatment, etc.

It is not uncommon for people with BPD to misuse alcohol or other substances. This is likely to make problems related to the disorder worse and to bring along its own set of problems. If this is an issue for the person close to you, it may also benefit this person, you and others around him or her if use is made of a support programme such as that provided by Alcoholics Anonymous.

How does BPD affect family and social life?

BPD is a challenge to relationships. It can be met with good communication and emotional support. The illness may affect the ability to relate to others in the family and in the wider social network for periods of time. This is particularly true when the person is experiencing an episode of mania or depression. It is important to know that relationship problems can be resolved through good communication, support and by working at problems over time. At times it can be helpful to see a family/couples therapist or to join a family support group in order to get a new or different perspective on the issues important to coping and general harmony in the family and wider social network.

Future prospects

The nature of BPD is such that a person with this diagnosis is likely to have ups and downs in the coming years, but that does not mean that there is any reason to lose hope for the future.

With the help of medication, therapy and generally supportive surroundings, mood fluctuations can occur less often and become less pronounced.

With help and support it is very possible to manage the disorder, go after and achieve regular goals in life just like any other person and it is possible to have a fulfilled family, social and work life in the years to come.

Session 4
worksheet 2

Attentive engagement

1 *Get your priorities straight.* If someone whom you rely on for support is asking you to attend to his or her concerns you should have a *very* good reason not to oblige.

2 *Indicate that you will give this moment and their concerns your full attention.* This should be done in a clear manner by, for instance, sitting down or suggesting that you should both sit down. This simple move shows that you are not about to leave and that this conversation is important to you.

3 *Use open body language.* For example, do not cross your arms or 'square up' by sitting too close and with shoulders directly forward. This can come across as being defensive or aggressive. Let your arms rest alongside your body/in your lap and sit a little sideways to the person you are speaking to. Only look away from the other person to aid a comfortable flow to the conversation; otherwise look at them.

4 *Check and ensure you understand what is said.* Engage and pay attention. At the same time, make sure that you *show* that you are engaged by asking questions to clarify and fully understand what the other person is feeling, believing and needing from you. This is not a time for debate. It is a time for you to understand the other person.

5 *Speak less, understand more.* Make sure you speak far less than the other person.

Example of attentive engagement

Person A: "I know that this is a bad time and that you need to go to work, but I really need to get our holiday sorted."

Person B [giving top priority to Person A's concerns]: "OK, I don't have to leave just yet, so let's talk about it. But do you mind if I make us a coffee? Let's sit down in the kitchen. It's a better place to talk."

Person A: "No problem, but I need some answers. I have to book time off from work. Everyone else is booking their holidays and if we don't get this sorted soon we won't be able to go anywhere. I need to know now! No more excuses." [Sits down in kitchen.]

Person B: "Fair enough; you're annoyed with me. You think I can't commit and am not paying attention. Am I right? Is that how you feel?"

Person A: "Yes, and I can feel myself becoming annoyed with you again now, because I have already asked you a million times about this holiday."

Person B: "Yes, I can see that it must be annoying. Did you think that we would not get around to discussing it at all?"

Person A: "I just get so frustrated, angry and worried about whether we can do things like a normal couple. And it concerns me to think about a future where little things like this are always going to be a problem."

Person B: "I can understand why you are concerned. Is it only the holiday? Or is it more general than that? I really want to know what you are thinking and feeling about these things so that we can try and plan a way out of it."

[Please note that this is a particular conversation that may seem artificial to you especially when written down, as above. You need to develop and use your own words and style of attentive engagement. Remember: practice makes perfect.]

Session 4
worksheet 3

Managing the workplace

- Tick the box if you think this would benefit you in your current job.
- Put an E next to the box if you believe your employer would agree to it.
- Put an A next to the box if you intend to approach your employer about this.

Work structure:

☐ Working same hours every week.
☐ Working from home (fully or partly).
☐ Saying no to overtime.
☐ Part-time or reduced hours rather than full-time employment.
☐ Avoiding shift work.

Add your own examples:

_____
_____
_____
_____
_____
_____

Strategies with potential benefits for mood stability:

☐ Working with others, so blame and credit will be shared and not down to you alone.
☐ Working in an inviting environment with low stimuli (minimise noise, and work in an uncrowded, uncluttered room, etc.).
☐ Saying no to activities or aspects of the job that have acted as triggers for illness episodes in the past (check list from sessions two and three).
☐ Taking regular and frequent breaks during the day.

Add your own examples:

_____
_____
_____
_____
_____
_____

When not able to work:

☐ Being allowed the freedom to work back time used for mental health appointments at another time.
☐ Being allowed to leave work when you spot the signs of a relapse emerging.

Add your own examples:

_____
_____
_____
_____
_____
_____

Communication with your employer:

☐ Knowing what your employer is thinking about your job performance.
☐ Knowing what your employer is thinking about BPD.
☐ Having an appraisal system based on general performance rather than on punctuality and number of hours completed every month.

Add your own examples:

_____
_____
_____
_____
_____
_____

As   **Date when I will approach my employer**

_____   _____
_____   _____
_____   _____
_____   _____
_____   _____
_____   _____

Appendix A

Typical signs of depression

- Hopelessness
- Feeling as if he/she is no use to anyone
- Stopped caring about daily life
- Sleeps too much
- Cannot sleep
- No energy
- Sad (often worse in morning and a little better in the evening)
- Anxious or scared
- Irritable and short-fused
- Feeling empty
- Feeling guilty without any reasonable cause (free-floating guilt)
- Dislike of oneself or lack of self-esteem
- Concentration difficulties
- Feeling unattractive
- Lost the ability to experience pleasure
- Being easily angered
- Dislike of socialising
- Seeking solitude
- Feeling burdened with 'the weight of the world'
- As if everything is grey or black
- Pain in head, back, stomach or other body-part
- Wanting to be dead
- Loss of emotions ('hollow'/'empty')
- Extremely tired
- Loss of interest
- Motivation to do anything has gone
- Feeling slowed down
- Every little task is a major job
- Neglects personal hygiene
- Attitude to others becomes sarcastic or negative
- Feeling lonely even when not
- Internal explanations to problems: "It is all my fault"
- Global explanations to problems: "I'm useless at everything"
- Stable explanations to problems: "It will never change"
- Often tearful
- Feeling like a child that cannot impact on own life
- Feeling that others would be better off if he/she did not exist
- Believing that his or her life has been a failure
- Believing that others are out to get him or her (paranoid)
- Ruminations regarding past mistakes
- Loss of appetite or overeating
- Feeling physically sick/nausea
- Being constipated or having diarrhoea

Appendix B

Typical mania-related signs and statements made by clients about mania

- Full of hope for a truly *great* future
- Feeling as if the world is at his/her feet
- Thinking that everyone believes he/she is fantastic at everything
- Sleeps very little compared to the usual need
- Feels full of energy
- Experiences restlessness much of the time
- Annoyed that others are so slow at what they do
- He/she gets angry more easily
- He/she eats a lot more than average
- Thoughts of being superior to others
- Laughing a lot and for no good reason without being able to stop
- Having a sense of things, people or oneself being 'unreal'
- Creating a lot of plans
- Concentration difficulties
- Difficulties completing tasks
- Engaging in multiple tasks at once
- Extremely ambitious in plans with high expectations for the outcome
- Feeling very creative
- Sense of time distorted (slowed down or speeded up)
- Being very impatient
- Thoughts are very clear
- Greater need for socialising
- Annoyed that others cannot see his/her 'greatness'
- Belief that he/she has special powers (foresee future, solve the world's problems, etc.)
- Full of anxiety
- Getting a lot of 'strange' or 'bizarre' ideas
- Experiencing that hearing and/or sight is improved
- Feeling a pressure to write
- Feeling a pressure to speak
- Engaging in dangerous activity (reckless driving, etc.)
- Drinking more alcohol than usual
- Showing poor judgement
- Spending a lot of money (spending sprees)
- Spending or investing a lot of money on things not really needed
- Feeling the body temperature go up ('flushed')
- Sexually very active or engaging in risky sexual practices or sexual practices not usually engaged in
- Being very productive
- Believing he/she has a special role in the world/world history
- Believing that others are out to

get him/her (paranoid)
- Showing no consideration for other peoples' needs
- Friends or family start to notice that he/she has changed

- He/she experiences friends and family as being overly critical
- Lots of thoughts going through his/her head at any one time

References

Bauer, M.S. and McBride, L., *Structured Group Psychotherapy for Bipolar Disorder. The Life Goals Program*, New York, Springer Publishing Company, 1996

Beck, A.T., Weissman, A., Lester, D. and Trexler, L., 'The measurement of pessimism: The Hopelessness Scale', *Journal of consulting psychology*, Vol. 42, 1974. pp.861-5

Coryell, W., Scheftner, W., Keller, M., Endicott, J., Maser, J. and Klerman, G.L., 'The enduring psychosocial consequences of mania and depression', *American Journal of Psychiatry*, Vol. 150, 1993. pp.720–7

Dion, G.L., Tohen, M., Anthony, W.A. and Waternaux, C.S., 'Symptoms and functioning of patients with bipolar disorder six months after hospitalization', *Hospital and Community Psychiatry*, Vol. 39, 1988. pp.652–7

Ehlers, C.L., Frank, E. and Kupfer, D.J., 'Social zeitgebers and biological rhythms: A unified approach to understanding the aetiology of depression', *Archives of General Psychiatry*, Vol. 45, 1988. pp.948–52

Fromm-Reichman, F., 'Intensive psychotherapy of manic-depressives: a preliminary report', *Confina Neurologica*, Vol. 9, 1949. pp.158–65

Geddes, J.R., Burgess, S., Hawton, K., Jamison, K. and Guy, M., 'Long-term Lithium Therapy for Bipolar Disorder: Systemic Review and Meta-analysis of Randomized Controlled Trials', *American Journal of Psychiatry*, Vol. 161, 2004. pp.217–22

Gitlin, M.J., Swendsen, J., Heller, T.L. and Hammen, C., 'Relapse and impairment in bipolar disorder', *American Journal of Psychiatry*, Vol. 152 (11), 1995. pp.1635–40

Goodwin, F.K. and Jamison, K.R., *Manic Depressive Illness*, New York, Oxford University Press, 1990

Greenhouse, W.J., Meyer, B. and Johnson, S.L., 'Coping and medication adherence in bipolar disorder', *Journal of Affective Disorders*, Vol. 59, 2000. pp.237–41

Huxley, N.A., 'Beyond medication: Taking a new look at psychosocial treatments for Bipolar Disorder' in Maj, M., Akiskal, H.S., Lopez-Ibor, J.J. and Sartorius, N. (eds.), *Bipolar Disorder*, Vol. 5, 2002, in WPA Series Evidence and Experience in Psychiatry, Chichester, John Wiley and Sons Ltd

Johnson, S.L., Sandrow, D., Meyer, B., Winters, R., Miller, I., Keitner, G. and Solomon, D., 'Life events involving goal-attainment and the emergence of manic symptoms', *Journal of Abnormal Psychology*, Vol. 109, 2000. pp.721–7

Keck, P.E., McElroy, S.L., Strakowski, S.M., Bourne, M.L. and West, S.A., 'Compliance with maintenance treatment in bipolar disorder', *Psychopharmacology Bulletin*, Vol. 33, 1997. pp.87–91

Kessler, R.C., Rubinow, D.R., Holmes, C., Abelson, J.M. and Zhao, S., 'The epidemiology of DSM-III-R bipolar disorder in a general population survey', *Psychological Medicine*, Vol. 27, 1997. pp.1079–89

Lam, D.H., Watkins, E.R., Hayward, P., Bright, J., Wright, K., Kerr, N., Parr-Davis, G. and Sham, P., 'A randomized controlled study of cognitive therapy for relapse prevention for bipolar affective disorder', *Archives of General Psychiatry*, Vol. 60, 2003. pp.145–52

Michalak, E.E., Yatham, L.N. and Lam, R.W., 'The Role of Psychoeducation in the Treatment of Bipolar Disorder: A Clinical Perspective', *Clinical Approaches in Bipolar Disorders*, Vol. 3, 2004. pp.5–11

Miklowitz, D.J., *The Bipolar Survival Guide. What you and your family need to know*, London, The Guilford Press, 2002

Miklowitz, D.J. and Goldstein, M.J., *Bipolar disorder: A family-focused treatment approach*, New York, The Guilford Press, 1997

Nilsson, A., 'Lithium Therapy and Suicide Risk', *Journal of Clinical Psychiatry*, Vol. 60 (2), 1999. pp.85–8

Scott, J. and Todd, G., 'Is There a Role for Psychotherapy in Bipolar Disorders?', *Clinical Approaches in Bipolar Disorders*, Vol. 1, 2002. pp.22–30

Seligman, M.E.P., 'Depression and learned helplessness' in Friedman, R.J. and Katz, M.M. (eds.), *The Psychology of Depression: Contemporary Theory and Research*, New York, John Wiley and Sons Ltd, 1974

Seligman, M.E.P., *Helplessness: On Depression, Development and Death*, San Francisco, Freeman Publications, 1975

Sorensen, J., *A Longitudinal Study of Bipolar Disordered Clients Going Through an Intensive Psycho-educational Intervention Programme*, Unpublished Doctoral Thesis, University of Hertfordshire, 2004

Sorensen, J., Done, D.J. and Rhodes, J., 'The development and evaluation of a novel, brief psycho-educational and cognitive therapy for bipolar disorder: The Sorensen Therapy for Instability in Mood', *Behavioural and Cognitive Psychotherapy* (submitted)

Tohen, M., Carlos, A., Zarate, Jr., Hennen, J., Hari-Mandir, K.K., Strakowski, S.M., Gebre-Medhin, P., Salvatore, P. and Baldessarini, R.J., 'The McLean-Harvard First Episode Mania Study, Prediction of Recovery and First Recurrence', *American Journal of Psychiatry*, Vol. 160, 2003. pp.2099–107

Torrey, E.F. and Knable, M.B., *Surviving Manic Depression. A manual on bipolar disorder for patients, families and providers*, New York, Basic Books, 2002

Zubin, J. and Spring, B., 'Vulnerability – A New View of Schizophrenia', *Journal of Abnormal Psychology*, Vol. 86 (2), 1977. pp.103–26